THE MATERNAL JOURNAL

A personal record of my pregnancy

To Marijo
Ruth Wolfe

by
Linda Schwartz
Carolyn McWilliams Bogad
Ruth Meiselman Wolfe

Published and distributed by
Woodbridge Press Publishing Company
Post Office Box 6189
Santa Barbara, California 93111

Library of Congress Cataloging in Publication Data
Schwartz, Linda.
    The maternal journal.
    1. Pregnancy—Forms. 2. Medical records—Forms.
I. McWilliams Bogad, Carolyn. II. Meiselman Wolfe, Ruth.
III. Title.
RG525.S3974   618.3'4   82-4736
ISBN 0-912800-99-2   AACR2

THIS IS A JOURNAL OF MY EXPERIENCES, THOUGHTS
AND FEELINGS DURING MY PREGNANCY WITH
_____ WHO WAS BORN ON:

‾‾‾‾, ‾‾‾‾‾, ‾‾‾‾,
day   month   year,

_____
signature

_____
date

Dedicated to:
Stephen, Michael, Lesley, Molly, Neely
Heather, Geoffrey, and Erin
—who continually surprise us with their ability
to enrich our lives.

TABLE OF CONTENTS

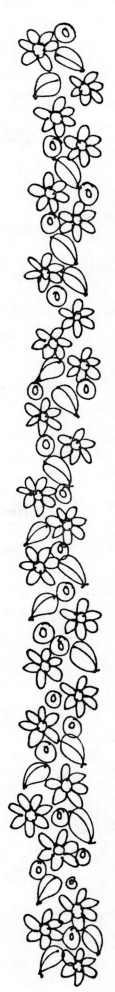

Page

First Trimester: A Time of Discovery.......................1

    Discovery Day...........................2

    Pictures of Me..........................3

    Medical Matters.........................4

    Office Visits.........................5—11

    Office Visits: The Final Lap..........12—15

    Famous Last Words.......................16

    What's Happening........................17

    Sibling Views...........................18

    Worthwhile Reading......................19

    Found: The Perfect Mother...............20

    Help Wanted.............................21

    Third Month Evaluation..................22

Second Trimester: A Time of Reflection.......23

    Heritage................................24

    Heritage, cont..........................25

    The Possibilities.......................26

    Personality Plus........................27

    Inheritances............................28

    Wishful Thinking........................29

    My Own Style............................30

    Changes in Me...........................31

    The Working Mother......................32

    What's in a Name?.......................34

    With a Little Help from My Friends......35

    Famous Firsts...........................36

    A Baby Contract.........................37

    Sixth Month Evaluation..................38

TABLE OF CONTENTS (continued)

Page

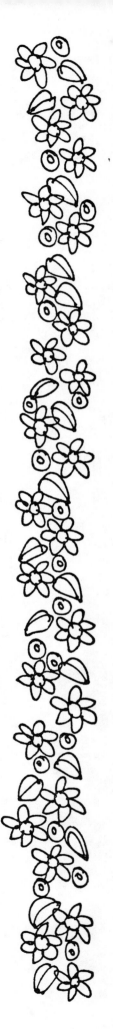

Third Trimester: A Time of Preparation.........................39

    Family Interviews.................................40

    A Space for Baby................................41

    For Nursing Mothers...........................42

    Prepared Childbirth Classes...................43

    Showers...44

    Special Favors to Remember..................45

    Ninth Month Only..............................46

    Innermost Thoughts...........................47

    All Set to Go...................................48

    Towards the End...............................49

    Special Reflections.........................50—51

    Ninth Month Evaluation.......................52

A Time for Change......................................53

    Labor Day.......................................54

    Blow-by-Blow Description of Birth..............55

    For Caesarean Mothers.......................56

    First Impressions...............................57

    Father's View....................................58

    After the Delivery...............................59

    My Own Experience........................60—61

    Homecoming Day..............................62

    Father's Reflections............................63

    Portraits of Baby...........................64—65

    Getting Acquainted with Baby.................66

    A Personality of His/Her Own.................67

    Reflections.................................68—69

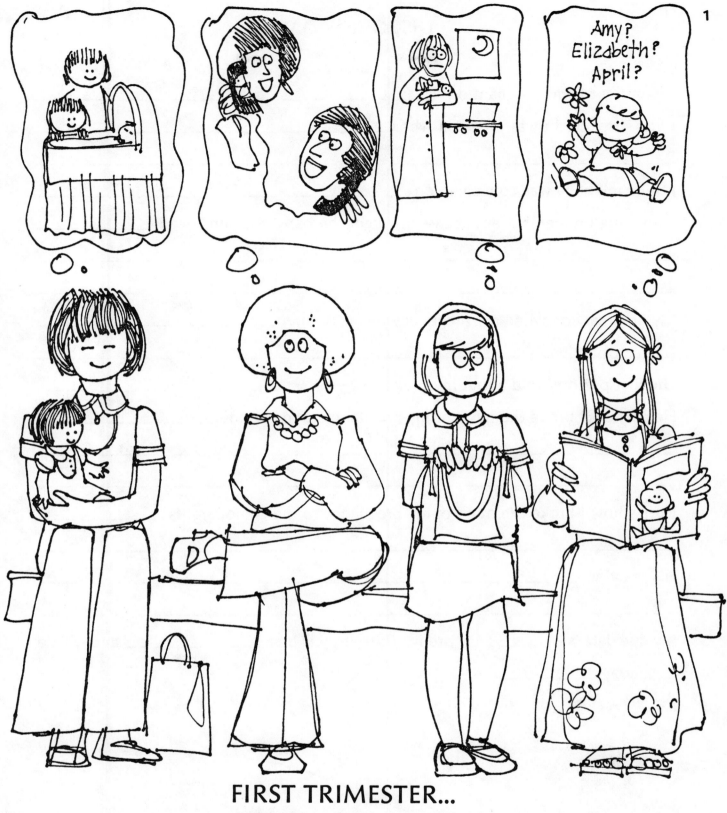

FIRST TRIMESTER...
A Time of Discovery

DISCOVERY DAY

I found out I was pregnant on _____

I first suspected I was pregnant when _____

_____

I think my baby was conceived on _____

One thing I remember about the day/night the baby was conceived _____

_____

_____

My first reaction when my pregnancy was confirmed_____

_____

The first person I told about my pregnancy was _____

Here's how I broke the news of my pregnancy to my partner_____

_____

_____

Here's how I broke the news of my pregnancy to the grandparents _____

_____

His reaction _____

_____

My due date is_____. I predict the baby will be a_____ and will be

____days_____.
  early-late

PICTURES OF ME

Who am I? At what point and from what perspective am I beginning this journey?

Write a brief description in each frame.

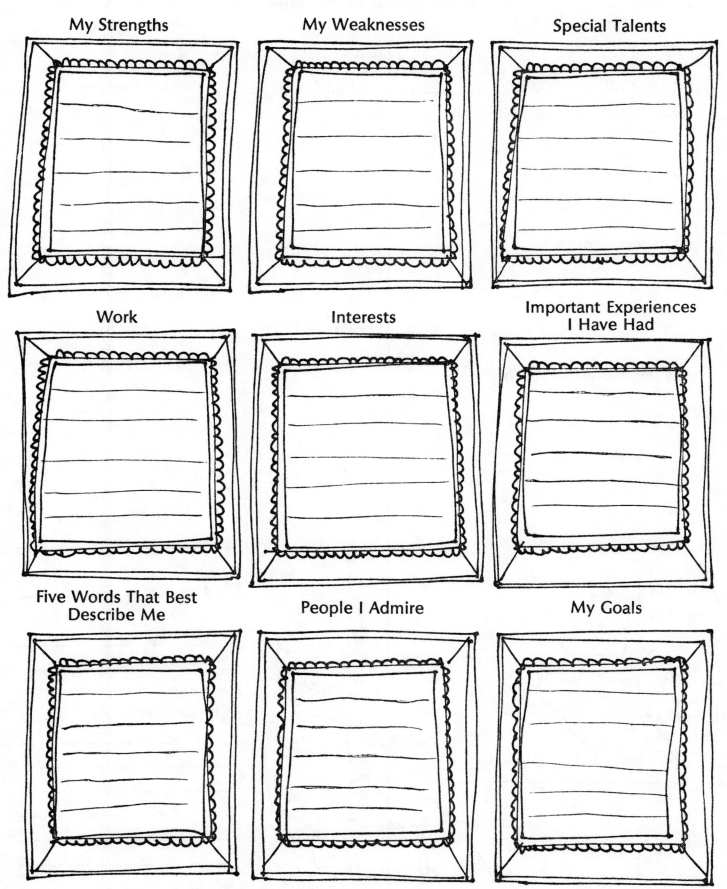

My Strengths

My Weaknesses

Special Talents

Work

Interests

Important Experiences I Have Had

Five Words That Best Describe Me

People I Admire

My Goals

MEDICAL MATTERS

I chose _____ for my medical care during my pregnancy.
My reasons for this choice:

My first office visit was _____ when I was _____ weeks pregnant.
The doctor's general philosophy and instructions:

My special concerns:

My feelings about this first visit:

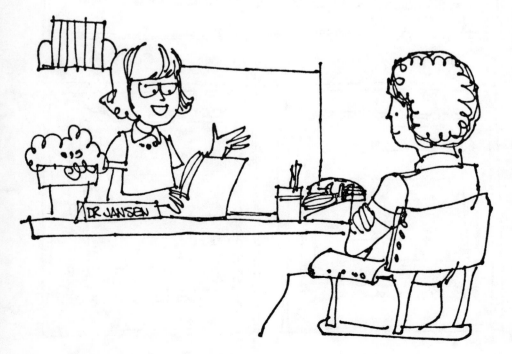

VITAL STATISTICS

Age_____

Weight _____

Blood type _____

General Health _____

_____

_____

Medical problems of conditions that

might affect this pregnancy _____

_____

_____

_____

_____

_____

_____

Due date _____

OFFICE VISITS

Date_____ _____weeks pregnant   weight_____

Questions and concerns:

Special instructions:

Reflections:

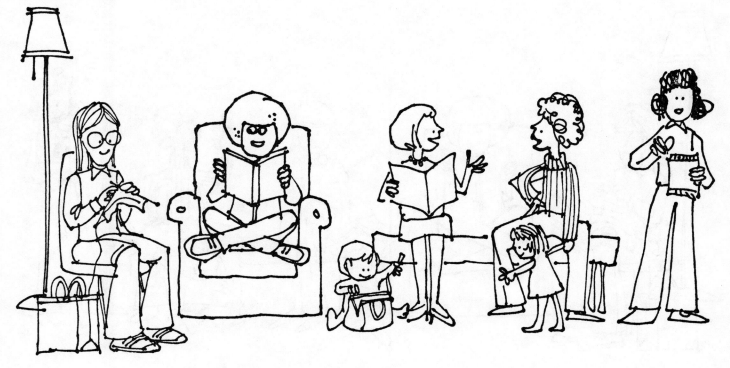

OFFICE VISITS

Date_____   _____weeks pregnant   weight_____

Questions and concerns:

Special instructions:

Reflections:

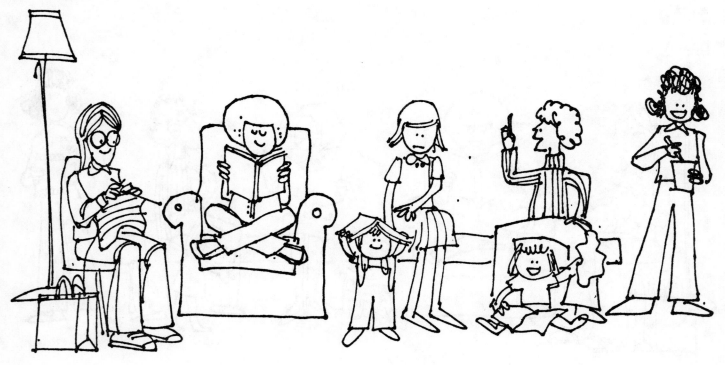

OFFICE VISITS

Date_____   _____weeks pregnant   weight_____

Questions and concerns:

Special instructions:

Reflections:

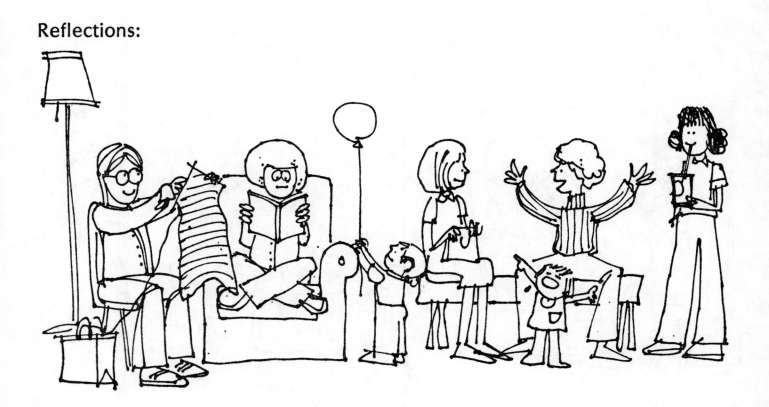

OFFICE VISITS

Date_____   _____weeks pregnant   weight_____

Questions and concerns:

Special instructions:

Reflections:

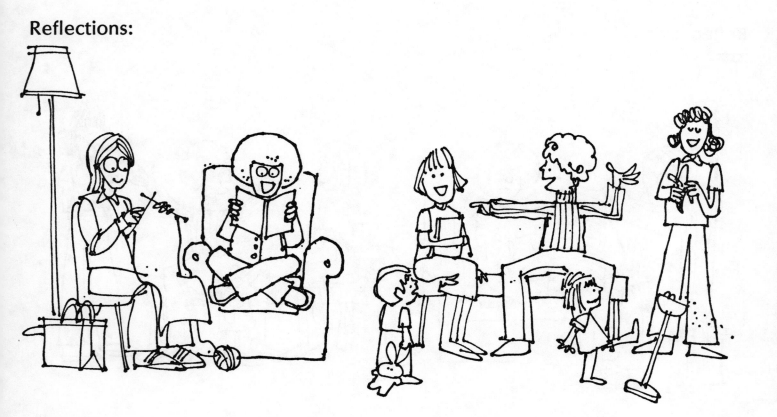

Date_____   _____weeks pregnant   weight_____

Questions and concerns:

Special instructions:

Reflections:

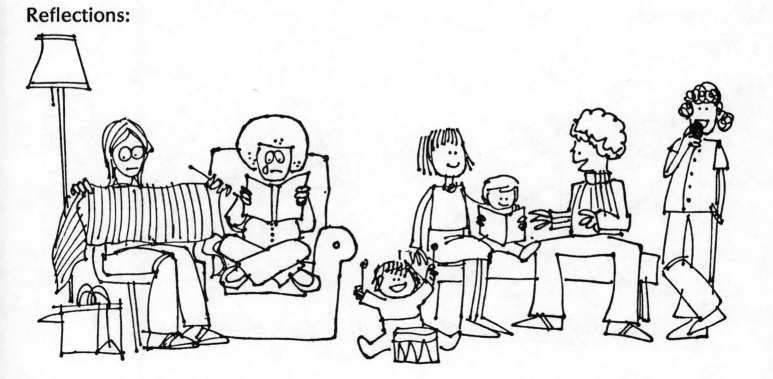

OFFICE VISITS

Date_____   _____weeks pregnant   weight_____

Questions and concerns:

Special instructions:

Reflections:

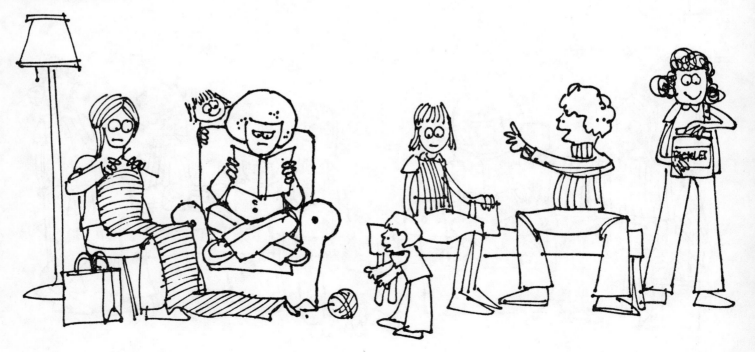

OFFICE VISITS

Date_____   _____weeks pregnant   weight_____

Questions and concerns:

Special instructions:

Reflections:

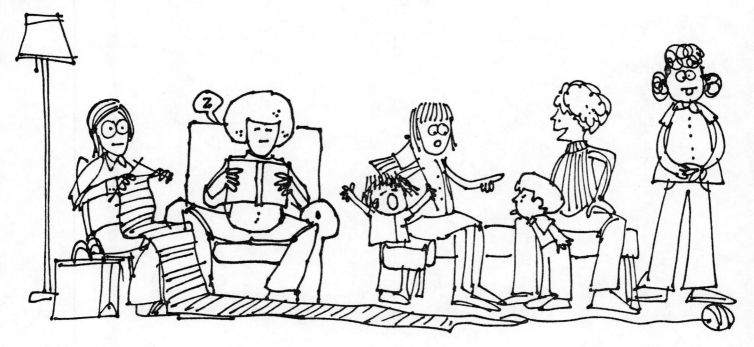

OFFICE VISITS—THE FINAL LAP

Date_____   _____weeks pregnant   weight_____

I am dilated _____cm.

Baby's heart rate_____

approximate size of baby_____

_____

Baby's position _____

_____

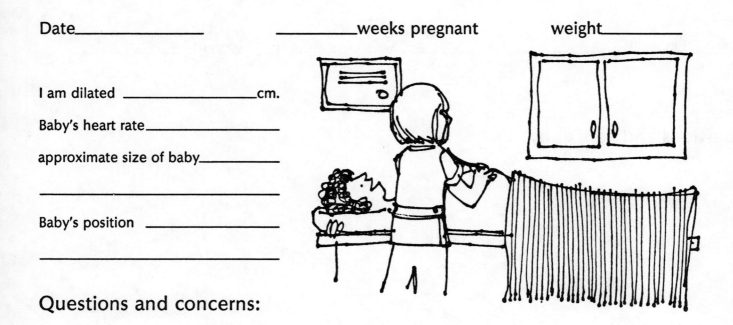

Questions and concerns:

Special instructions:

Reflections:

OFFICE VISITS—THE FINAL LAP

Date_____   _____weeks pregnant   weight_____

I am dilated _____cm.

Baby's heart rate_____

approximate size of baby_____

_____

Baby's position _____

_____

Questions and concerns:

Special instructions:

Reflections:

OFFICE VISITS—THE FINAL LAP

Date_____   _____weeks pregnant   weight_____

I am dilated _____cm.

Baby's heart rate_____

approximate size of baby_____

_____

Baby's position _____

_____

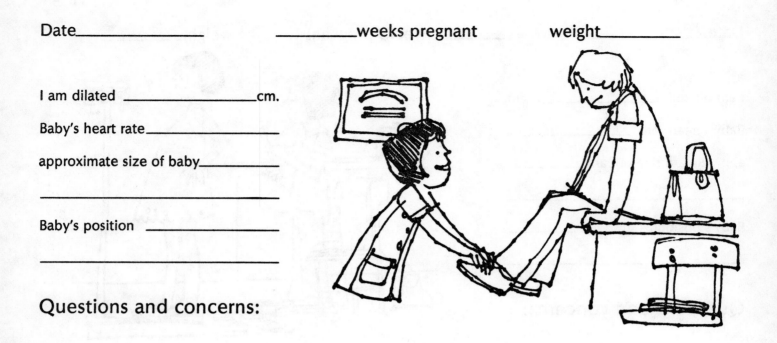

Questions and concerns:

Special instructions:

Reflections:

OFFICE VISITS—THE FINAL LAP

Date_____   _____weeks pregnant   weight_____

I am dilated _____cm.

Baby's heart rate_____

approximate size of baby_____

_____

Baby's position _____

_____

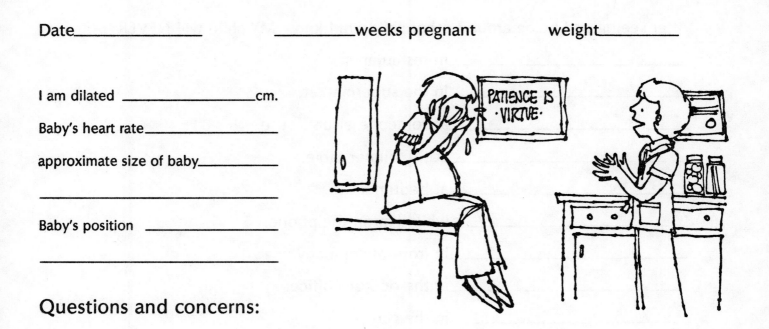

Questions and concerns:

Special instructions:

Reflections:

FAMOUS LAST WORDS

After seeing and being around other children, I know MY child will NEVER

_____in restaurants.

_____in the supermarket.

_____at someone else's house.

_____at the dinner table.

_____at bedtime.

_____while I'm on the phone.

_____in front of company.

_____at the doctor's office.

_____in the car.

_____in front of my mother-in-law.

_____while with the baby sitter.

_____in front of strangers.

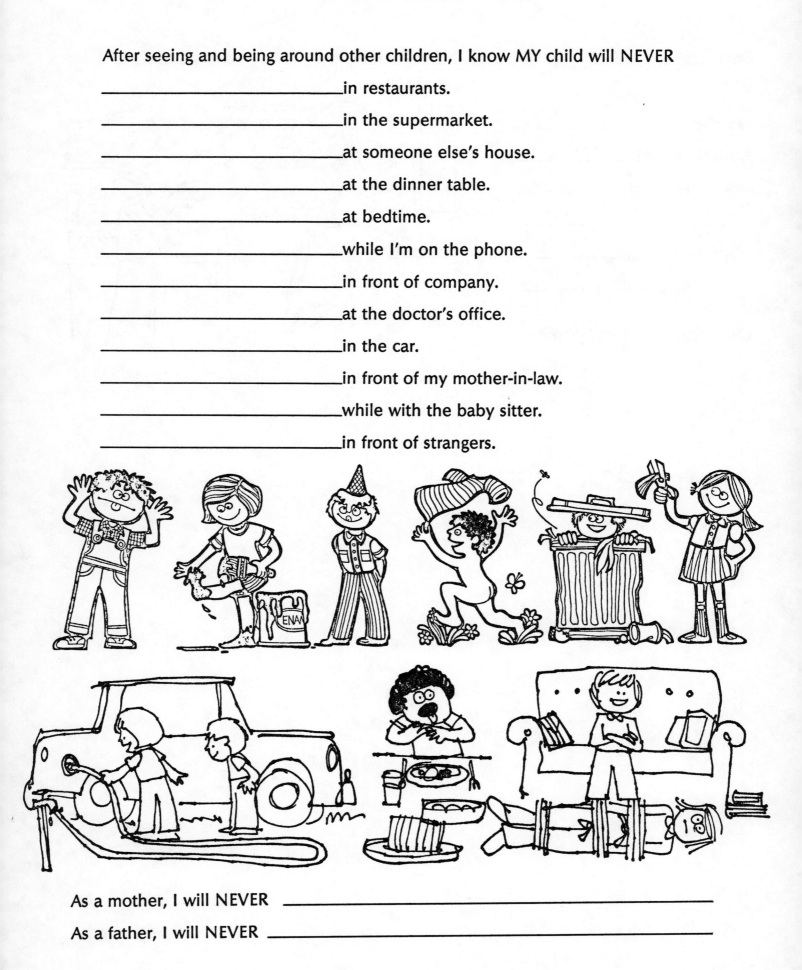

As a mother, I will NEVER _____

As a father, I will NEVER _____

WHAT'S HAPPENING

News items

People in the news

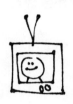

Fashion trends I'm seeing:

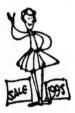

Fads

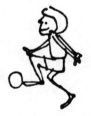

Music I'm listening to:

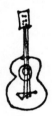

Sports

Books I'm reading:

My comments on the times:

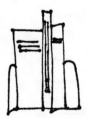

Hairstyles I'm seeing:

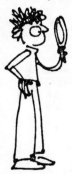

I have _____ children. Their ages are _____.

Here's how I told them about the baby.

Here's how I told them about pregnancy.

Their reactions and questions:

Here's what my children have to say about the baby:

One thing I plan to do to help with the baby _____

_____

One thing I refuse to do _____

_____

Something I'd like to teach the baby _____

_____

The best part about having a baby is _____

_____

The worst part about having a baby is _____

_____

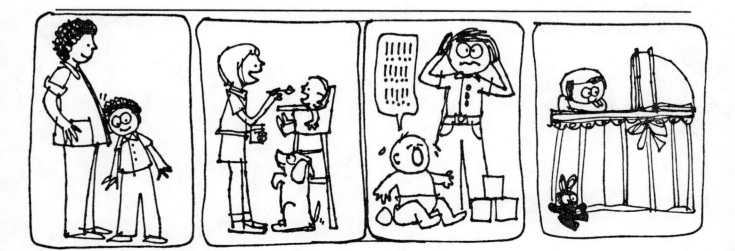

WORTHWHILE READING

Here are some books I read and found helpful during my pregnancy.

TITLE	AUTHOR	SUBJECT MATTER

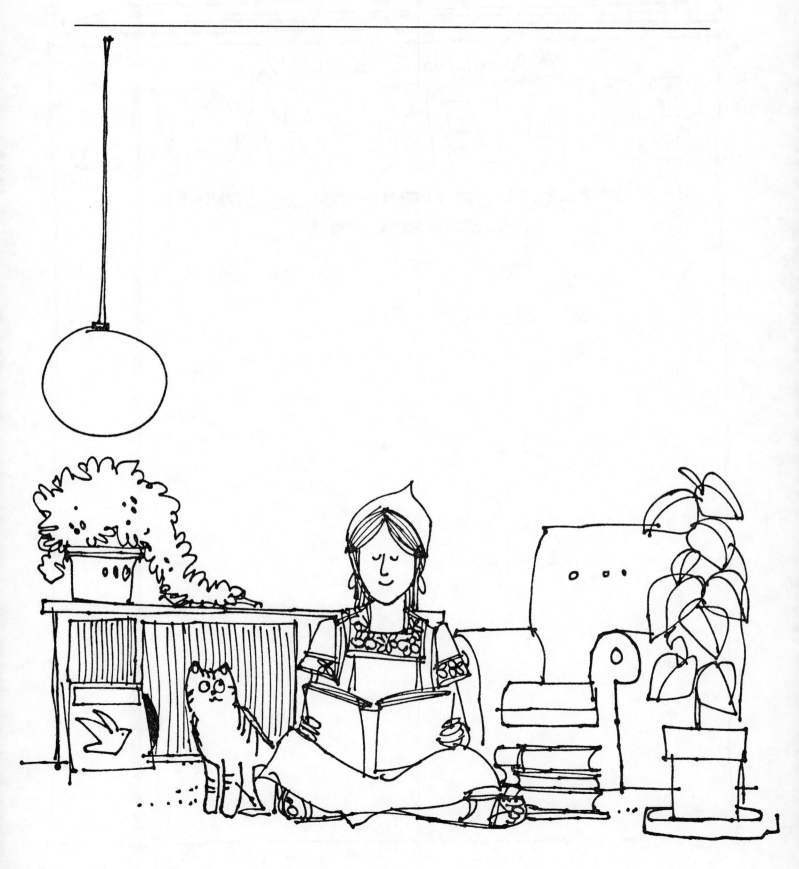

FOUND! THE PERFECT MOTHER!

Write an advertisement to sell yourself as a parent. Include all the great things you have going for you.

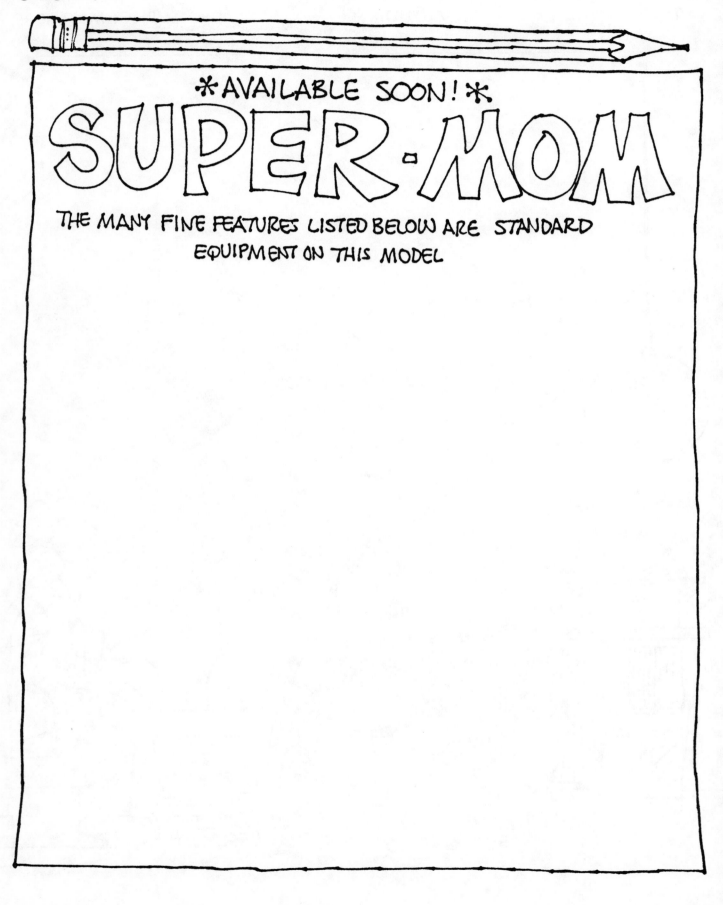

Write a "help wanted" ad to describe the trouble spots you might have as a parent.

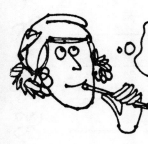

LET'S SEE.. I'LL NEED A BABY SITTER.. LATER ON A PIANO TEACHER... A GOOD SHOULDER TO CRY ON NOW AND THEN...

THIRD MONTH EVALUATION
(to be completed at the end of the first trimester)

1. My feelings about the way my body has changed: _____
_____
_____
_____
_____

2. My feelings towards my partner at this stage of my pregnancy: _____
_____
_____
_____
_____

3. My feelings about making love: _____
_____
_____
_____
_____

4. My feelings about having this baby: _____
_____
_____
_____

5. My partner's feelings about me and my pregnancy: _____
_____
_____
_____

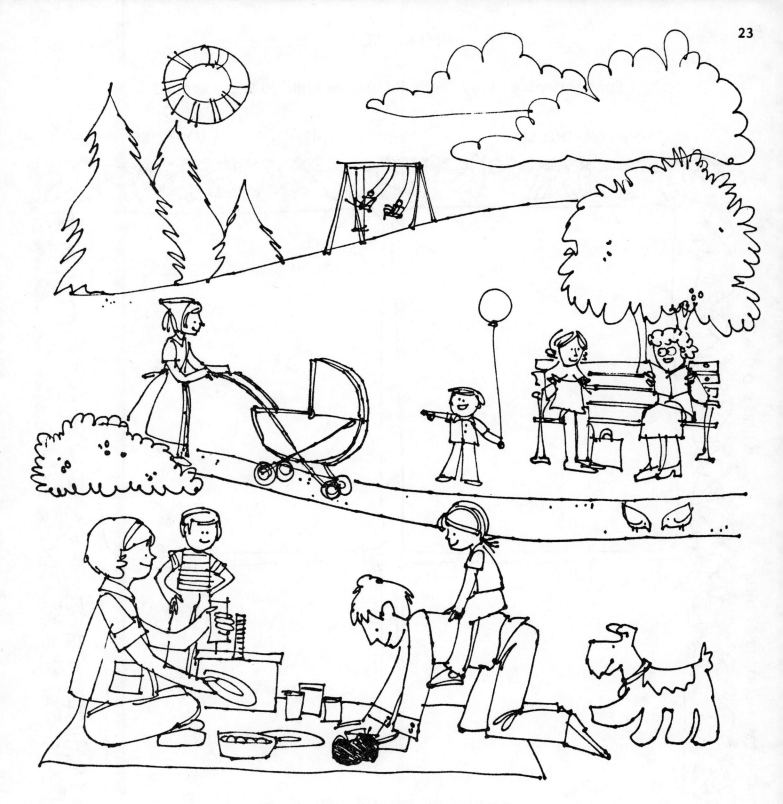

SECOND TRIMESTER...
a time for reflection

HERITAGE

Special people in my family I'd like my child to know about.

WHEN DID THEY LIVE?　　　　　　　WHAT DID THEY LOOK LIKE?

WHERE DID THEY LIVE?

WHAT ARE MY MEMORIES OF THEM?

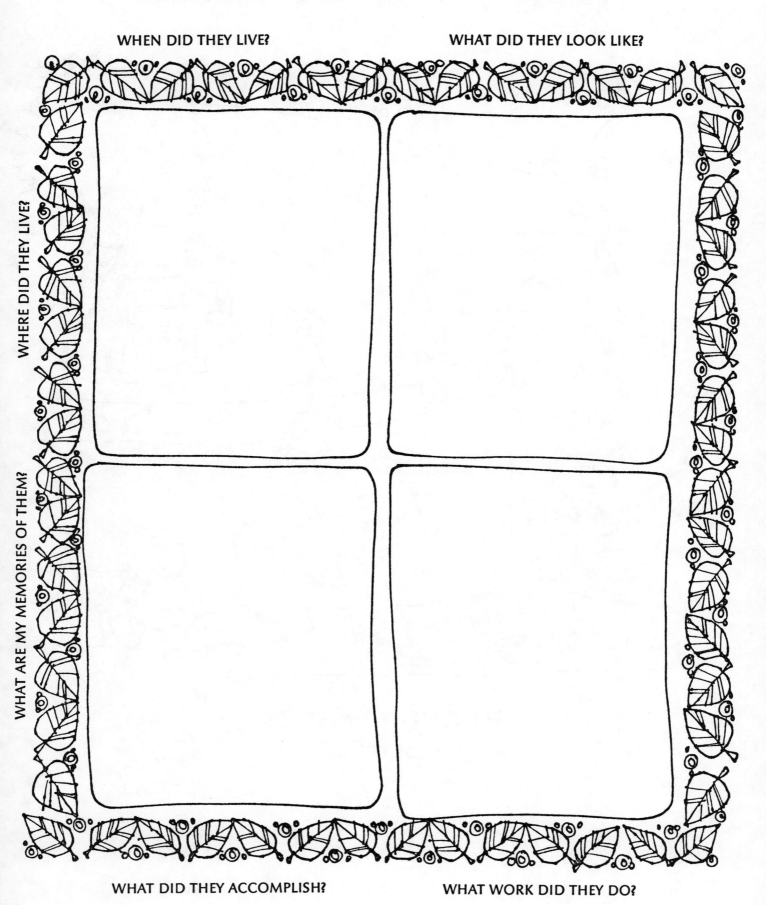

WHAT DID THEY ACCOMPLISH?　　　　　　WHAT WORK DID THEY DO?

HERITAGE

Special people in my husband's family I'd like my child to know about.

WHERE WERE THEY BORN?   WHAT MADE THEM SPECIAL?

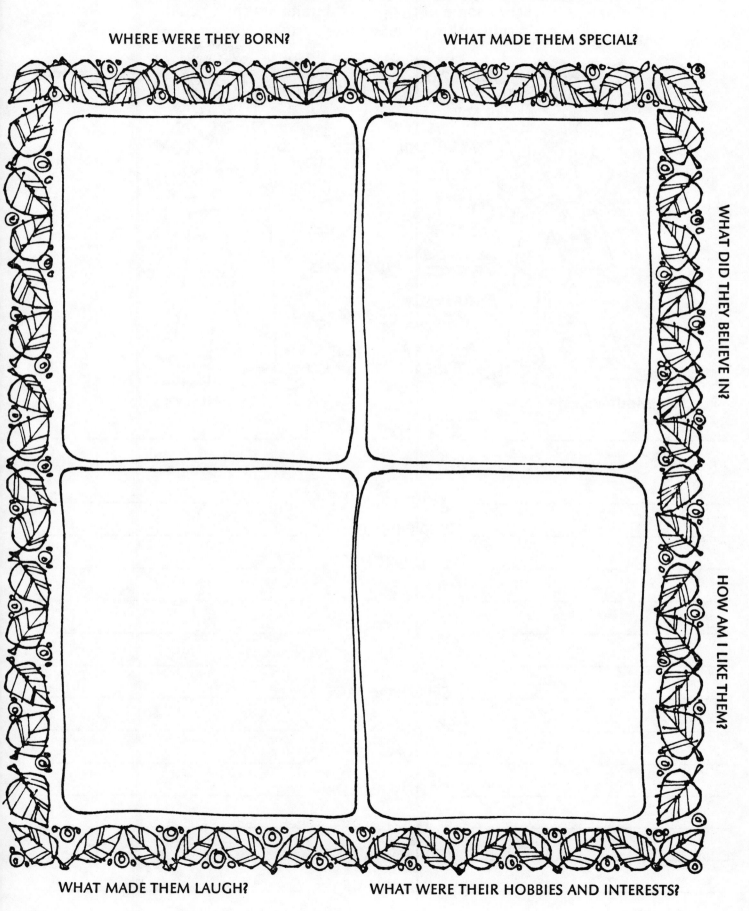

WHAT DID THEY BELIEVE IN?

HOW AM I LIKE THEM?

WHAT MADE THEM LAUGH?   WHAT WERE THEIR HOBBIES AND INTERESTS?

THE POSSIBILITIES

Here is a list of some of the physical traits my child could inherit from me and my partner.

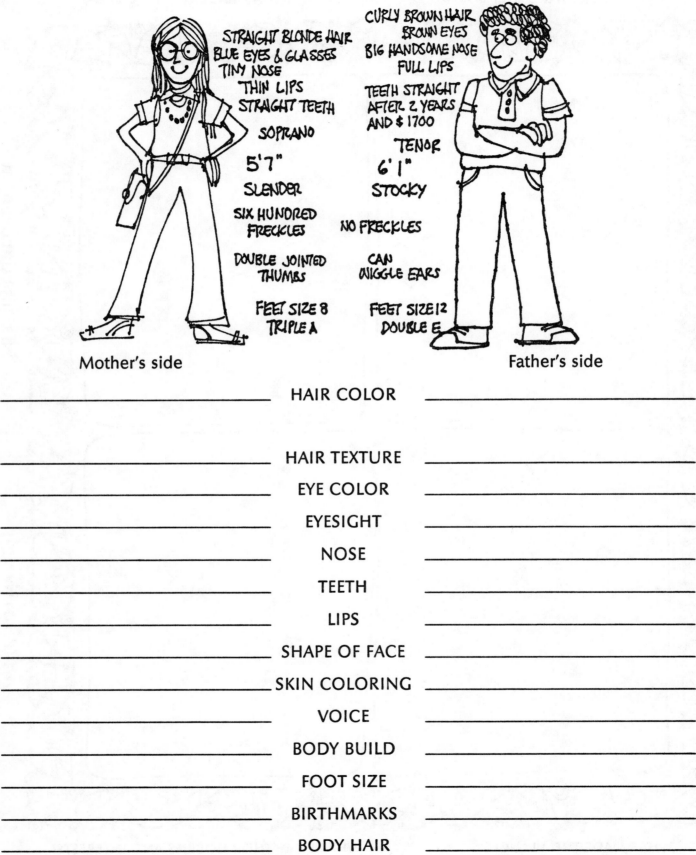

STRAIGHT BLONDE HAIR
BLUE EYES & GLASSES
TINY NOSE
THIN LIPS
STRAIGHT TEETH

SOPRANO

5'7"
SLENDER

SIX HUNDRED
FRECKLES

DOUBLE JOINTED
THUMBS

FEET SIZE 8
TRIPLE A

CURLY BROWN HAIR
BROWN EYES
BIG HANDSOME NOSE
FULL LIPS

TEETH STRAIGHT
AFTER 2 YEARS
AND $1700

TENOR

6'1"
STOCKY

NO FRECKLES

CAN
WIGGLE EARS

FEET SIZE 12
DOUBLE E

Mother's side

Father's side

_____ HAIR COLOR _____

_____ HAIR TEXTURE _____

_____ EYE COLOR _____

_____ EYESIGHT _____

_____ NOSE _____

_____ TEETH _____

_____ LIPS _____

_____ SHAPE OF FACE _____

_____ SKIN COLORING _____

_____ VOICE _____

_____ BODY BUILD _____

_____ FOOT SIZE _____

_____ BIRTHMARKS _____

_____ BODY HAIR _____

PERSONALITY PLUS

On a scale of one to ten, rate yourself and your partner in each of the categories below.

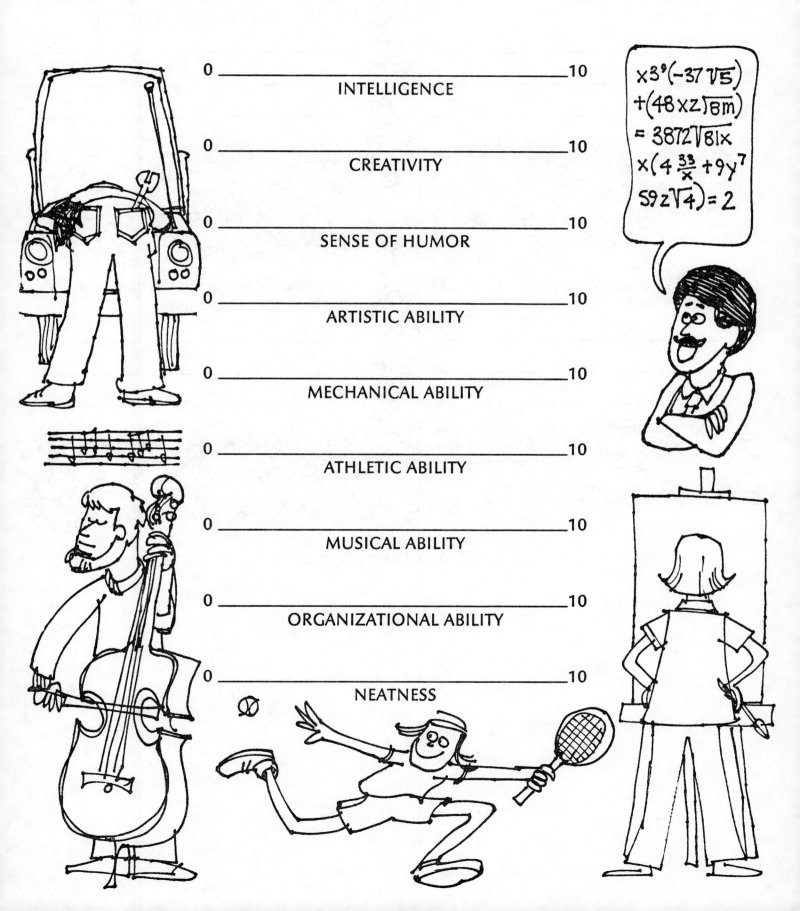

0 ——————————————— 10
INTELLIGENCE

0 ——————————————— 10
CREATIVITY

0 ——————————————— 10
SENSE OF HUMOR

0 ——————————————— 10
ARTISTIC ABILITY

0 ——————————————— 10
MECHANICAL ABILITY

0 ——————————————— 10
ATHLETIC ABILITY

0 ——————————————— 10
MUSICAL ABILITY

0 ——————————————— 10
ORGANIZATIONAL ABILITY

0 ——————————————— 10
NEATNESS

INHERITANCE

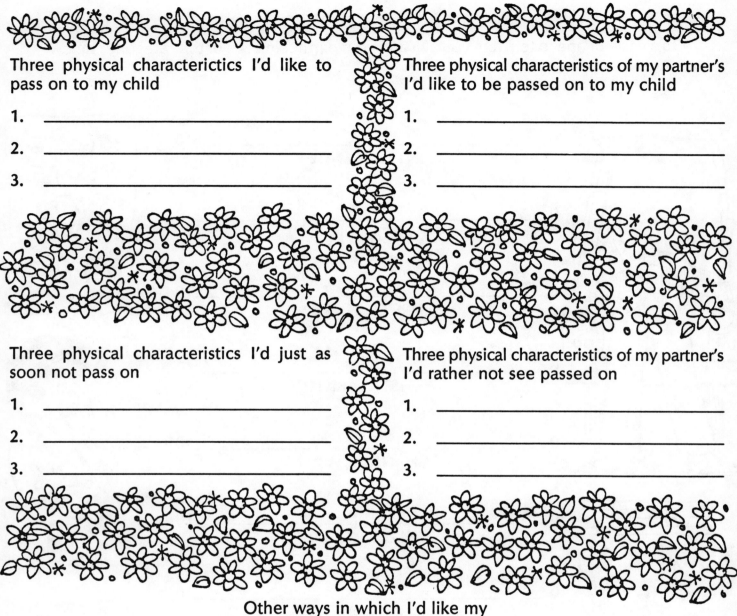

Three physical characterictics I'd like to pass on to my child

1. _____

2. _____

3. _____

Three physical characteristics of my partner's I'd like to be passed on to my child

1. _____

2. _____

3. _____

Three physical characteristics I'd just as soon not pass on

1. _____

2. _____

3. _____

Three physical characteristics of my partner's I'd rather not see passed on

1. _____

2. _____

3. _____

Other ways in which I'd like my
child to be like each of us

WISHFUL THINKING

3 values I would like to pass on to my child:

_____

_____

_____

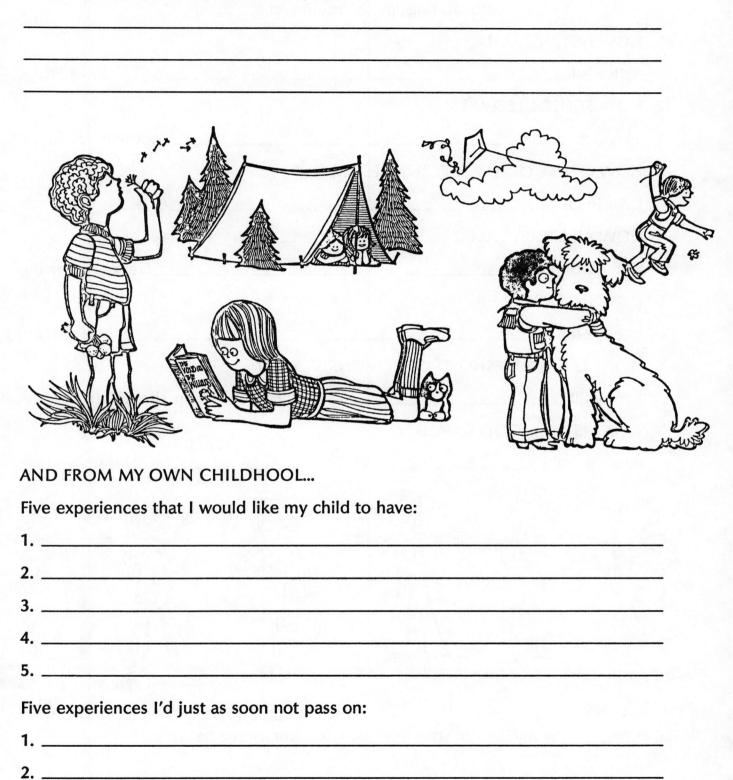

AND FROM MY OWN CHILDHOOL...

Five experiences that I would like my child to have:

1. _____

2. _____

3. _____

4. _____

5. _____

Five experiences I'd just as soon not pass on:

1. _____

2. _____

3. _____

4. _____

5. _____

DISCOVERING MY OWN STYLE

Mark an X on the continuum that best describes your own style.
No fair hugging the middle of the road!

1. HOW ACTIVE AM I?

Active Alice _____ Passive Paula

2. HOW SCHEDULED AM I?

Suzy Schedule _____ Spontaneous Sarah

3. HOW OPEN TO NEW EXPERIENCES AM I?

Dive In Dinah _____ Check It Out Opal

4. HOW ADAPTABLE AM I?

Flow With It Flow _____ Freak Out Freida

5. HOW INTENSE AM I?

Intense Ida _____ Mellow Molly

6. WHAT IS MY THRESHOLD OF RESPONSIVENESS?

Jumpy Jill _____ Sleep Through It All Sally

7. WHAT IS MY MOOD QUALITY?

Positive Polly _____ Negative Nelly

ACTIVE ALICE · CHECK IT OUT OPAL · POSITIVE POLLY · SUZY SCHEDULE · FREAK OUT FRIEDA · SLEEP THROUGH IT ALL SALI

REFLECTIONS

What strengths may my unique style give me in dealing with a baby?

What frustrations may I find because of my unique style?

CHANGES IN ME

Here is how pregnancy has affected

My diet:

My sleeping habits:

My work:

My moods:

My dreams:

My feelings about myself:

My relationships with others:

Some positive changes I
see in myself

Some negative changes I
see in myself

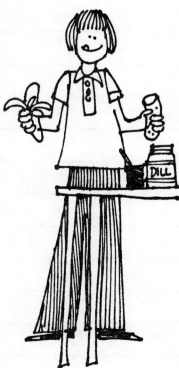

THE WORKING MOTHER

Description of my job _____

_____

_____

How I feel about my job _____

_____

I plan to work through my_____month of pregnancy.

I plan to return to work_____

_____

Some things I think I'll like about being home _____

_____

_____

_____

Reservations I have about being home _____

_____

_____

_____

What I will miss most when I stop working _____

_____

_____

What I won't miss when I stop working _____

_____

_____

MY PARTNER

Special things my partner has done for me during this pregnancy:

Things I wish he would do:

Things I wish he wouldn't do:

New things we've done together during my pregnancy:

Changes I see in him since I became pregnant:

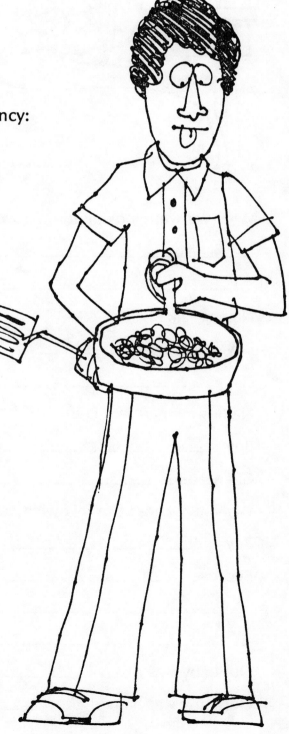

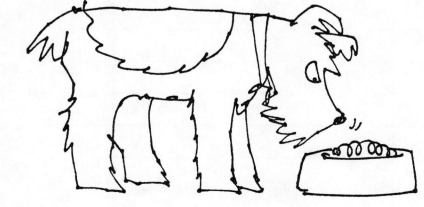

WHAT'S IN A NAME?

What we were looking for in a name _____

_____

_____

Names I liked:

Boy _____ _____ _____

Girl _____ _____ _____

Names my partner liked:

Boy _____ _____ _____

Girl _____ _____ _____

We finally chose the following names:

Boy _____ Girl _____

Because _____

_____

_____

Our baby was a _____ and was named _____

Our baby was named after _____

WITH A LITTLE HELP FROM MY FRIENDS

Special friends and how they have helped me during my pregnancy:

Family members and how they have helped:

Advice and ideas I got from others that I want to remember:

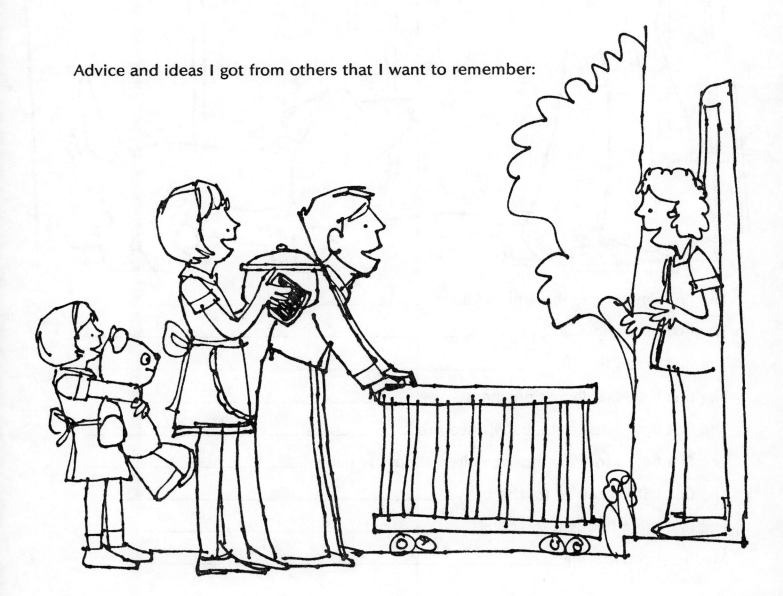

FIRSTS FOR ME

The first time I wore maternity clothes _____

The first maternity outfit I bought _____

The first time I felt life _____

The first time I really felt pregnant _____

The first time I heard the baby's heartbeat _____

The first time I told my other children about my baby _____

The first gift I received for the baby _____

The first thing I bought the baby _____

My first weird craving _____

A BABY CONTRACT

Here's who we have decided will:

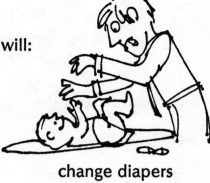

bathe the baby

_____

change diapers

_____

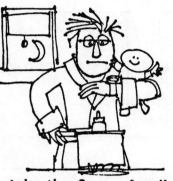

take the 2 a.m. feeding

_____

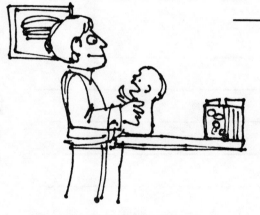

take baby to doctor

_____

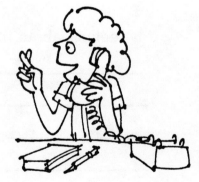

arrange for babysitter

_____

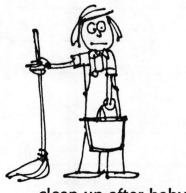

clean up after baby

_____

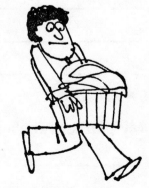

do baby's laundry

_____

SIXTH MONTH EVALUATION
(to be completed at the end of the second trimester)

1. My feelings about the way my body has changed: _____
_____
_____
_____
_____

2. My feelings towards my partner at this stage of my pregnancy: _____
_____
_____
_____
_____

3. My feelings about making love: _____
_____
_____
_____
_____

4. My feelings about having this baby: _____
_____
_____
_____

5. My partner's feelings about me and my pregnancy: _____
_____
_____
_____

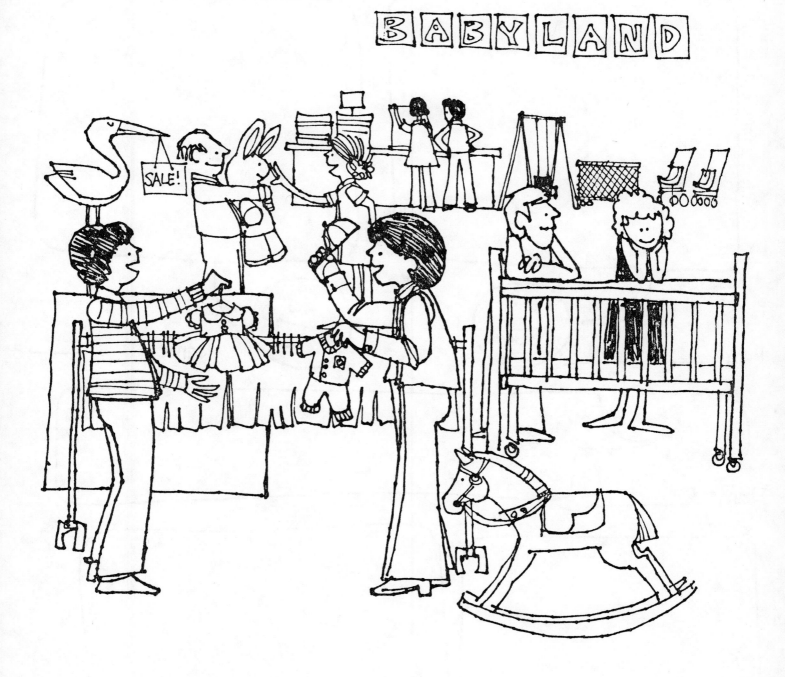

THIRD TRIMESTER...
A time of preparation

FAMILY INTERVIEWS
Here's what other family members have to say about the expected baby:

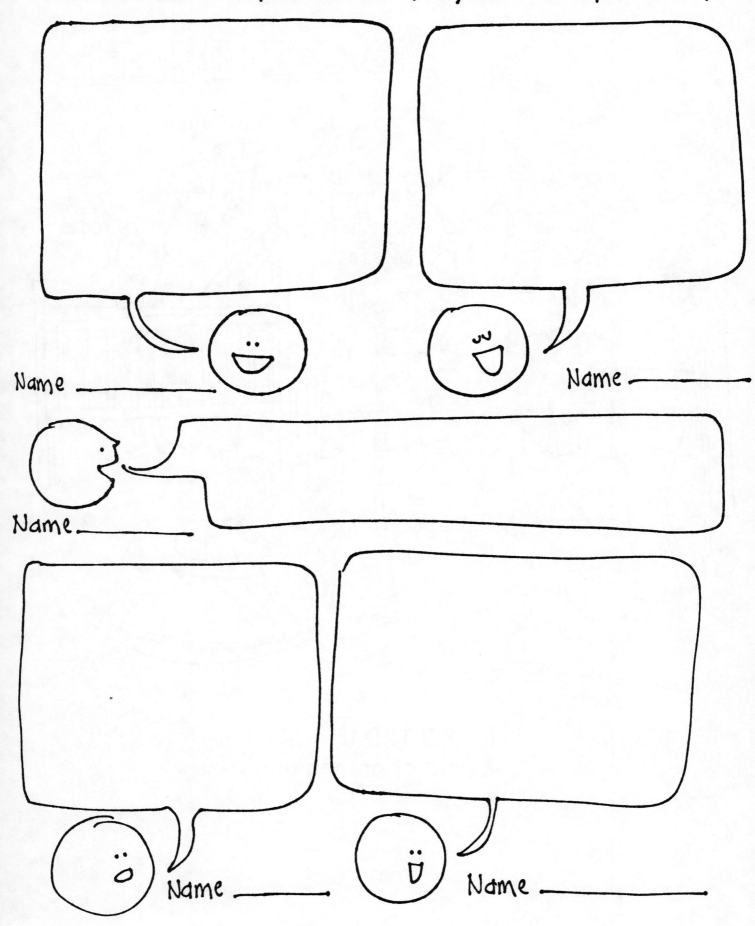

Name _____

Name _____

Name _____

Name _____

Name _____

A SPACE FOR BABY

When the baby comes home, his or her special place will be:

Things I have done to make the baby's space special:

I got some of my ideas from:

Other things I am making for the baby:

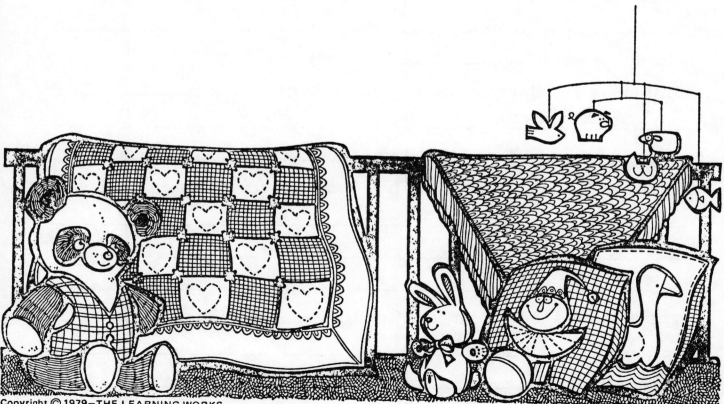

FOR NURSING MOTHERS

I decided to nurse my baby because _____

_____

_____

_____

_____

Some people who were influential in my decision to breastfeed were_____

_____

_____

I plan to nurse for about_____months.

I think I will especially enjoy nursing my baby because_____

_____

_____

Some advantages I think my baby will have because of breastfeeding: _____

_____

_____

_____

Some reservations I have about breastfeeding:_____

_____

_____

_____

PREPARED CHILDBIRTH CLASSES

I began prepared childbirth classes on _____

at _____

My instructor's name was: _____

Main topics covered each week in class:

week 1_____   week 4_____

week 2_____   week 5_____

week 3_____   week 6_____

My overall impression of the class: _____

_____

_____

My coach's overall impressions of the class: _____

_____

The classes have helped my most by _____

_____

I find it most convenient to practice_____

_____

Some interesting couples I met in class: _____

_____

_____

_____

SHOWERS

Here is a description of special showers and parties in honor of my expected baby. (You might want to include host or hostess, guests, gifts, food seved, special surprises, etc.)

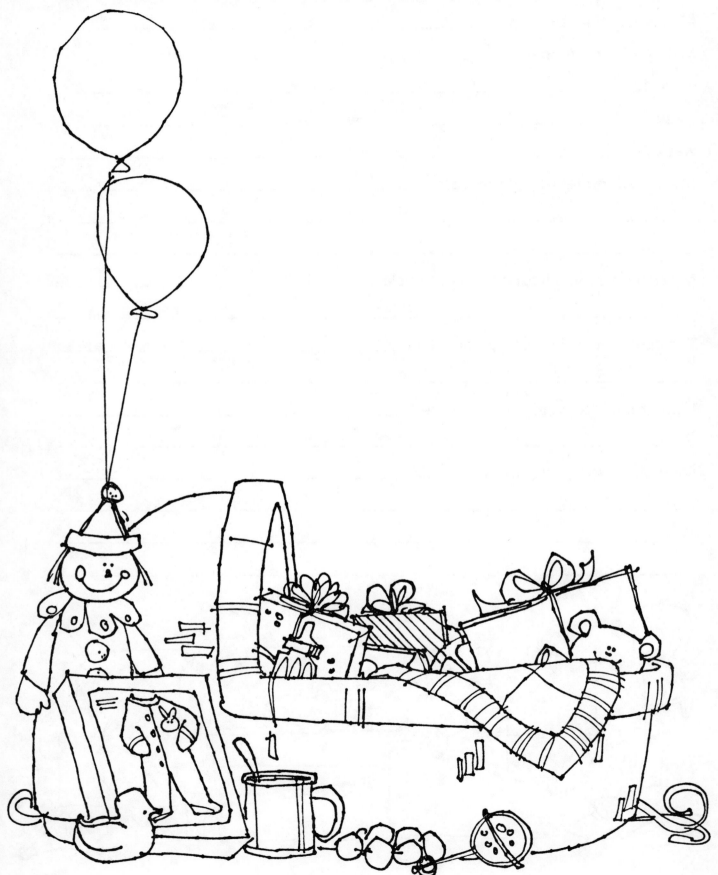

from

from

from

from

NINTH MONTH ONLY

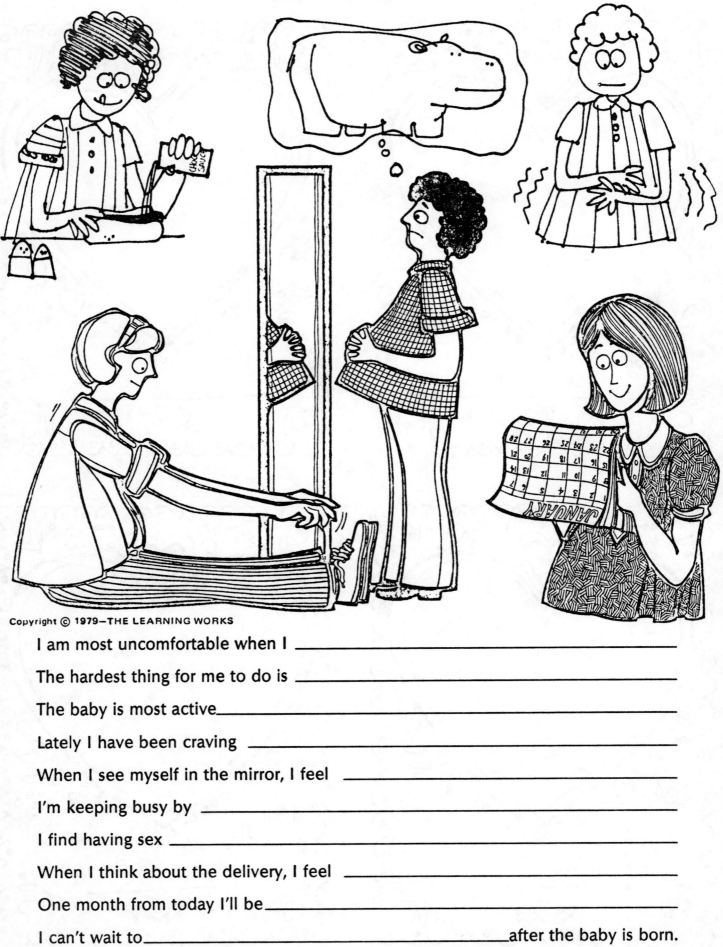

I am most uncomfortable when I _____

The hardest thing for me to do is _____

The baby is most active_____

Lately I have been craving _____

When I see myself in the mirror, I feel _____

I'm keeping busy by _____

I find having sex _____

When I think about the delivery, I feel _____

One month from today I'll be_____

I can't wait to_____after the baby is born.

INNERMOST THOUGHTS

The things that concern me most about the actual delivery are:_____

_____

_____

_____

_____

I think having a baby will add to my life by: _____

_____

_____

The things that concern me most about having a baby in my life are: _____

_____

_____

I think having a baby will affect my relationship with my partner by: _____

_____

_____

_____

I think having a baby will affect my other children by: _____

_____

_____

_____

ALL SET TO GO

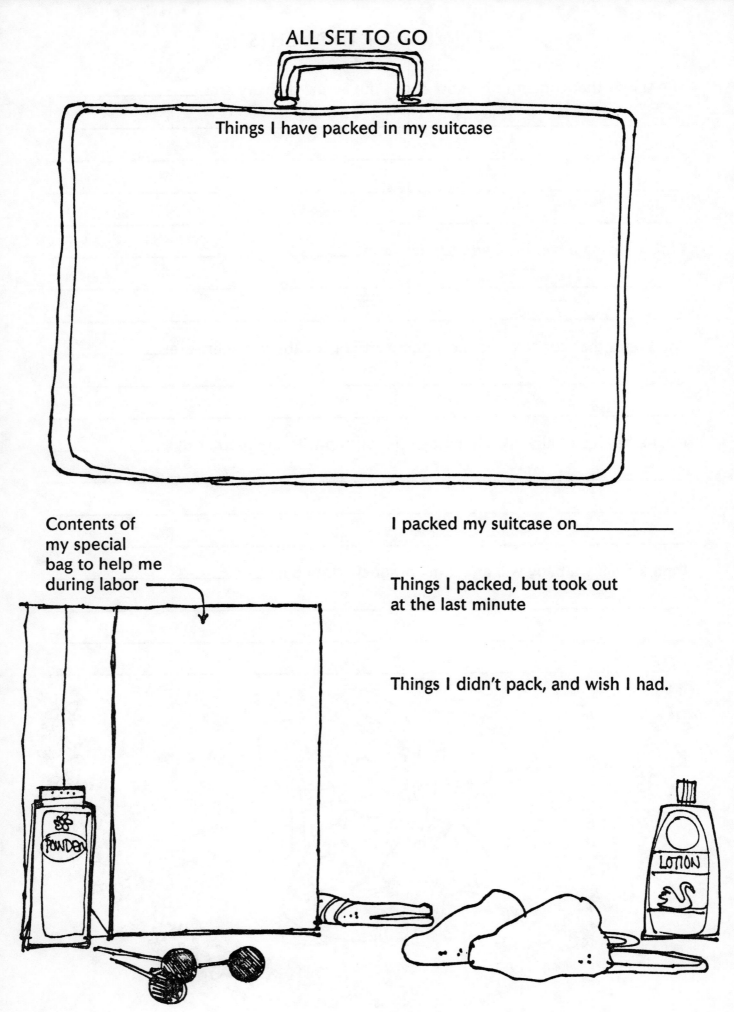

Things I have packed in my suitcase

Contents of
my special
bag to help me
during labor

I packed my suitcase on_____

Things I packed, but took out
at the last minute

Things I didn't pack, and wish I had.

TOWARDS THE END

The last advice I got from my mother _____
_____

The last advice I got from my mother-in-law _____
_____

The last time I slept through the night_____

The last time I could sleep on my stomach _____

The last time I felt sexy_____

The last time I could see my shoes while standing up _____

Some of the special things I did for myself during my last days of pregnancy _____

_____

_____

_____

_____

_____

_____

_____

_____

_____

SPECIAL REFLECTIONS DURING
MY LAST DAYS OF PREGNANCY

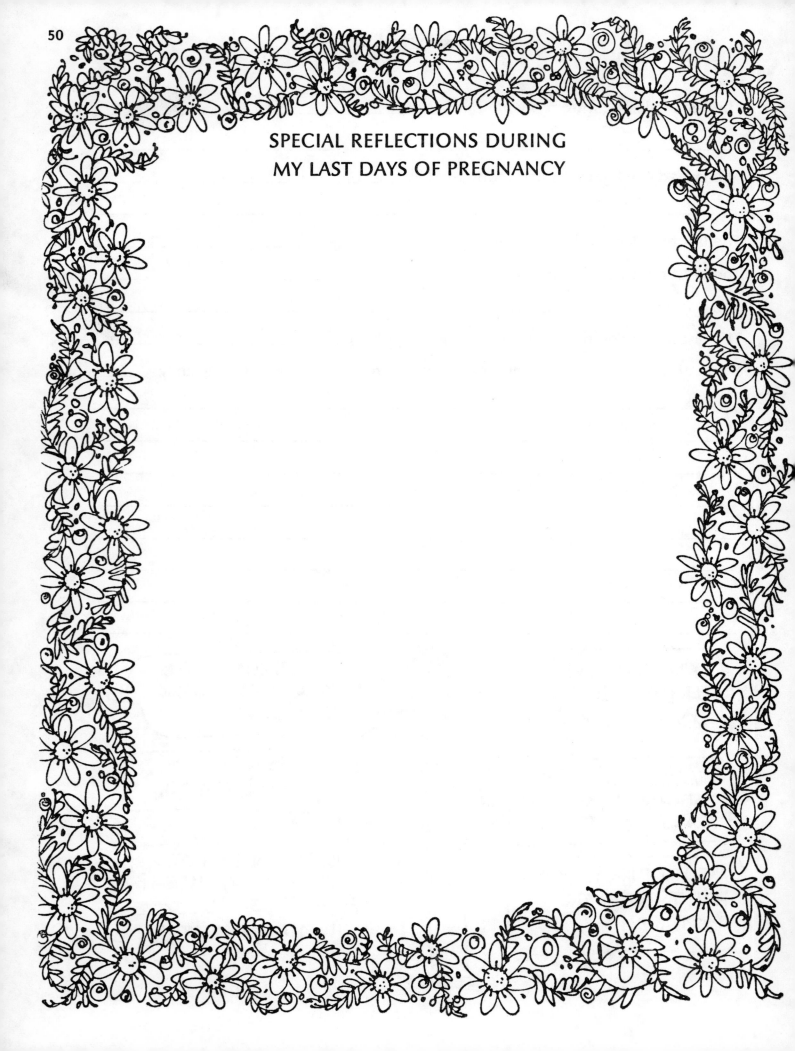

SPECIAL REFLECTIONS DURING
MY LAST DAYS OF PREGNANCY

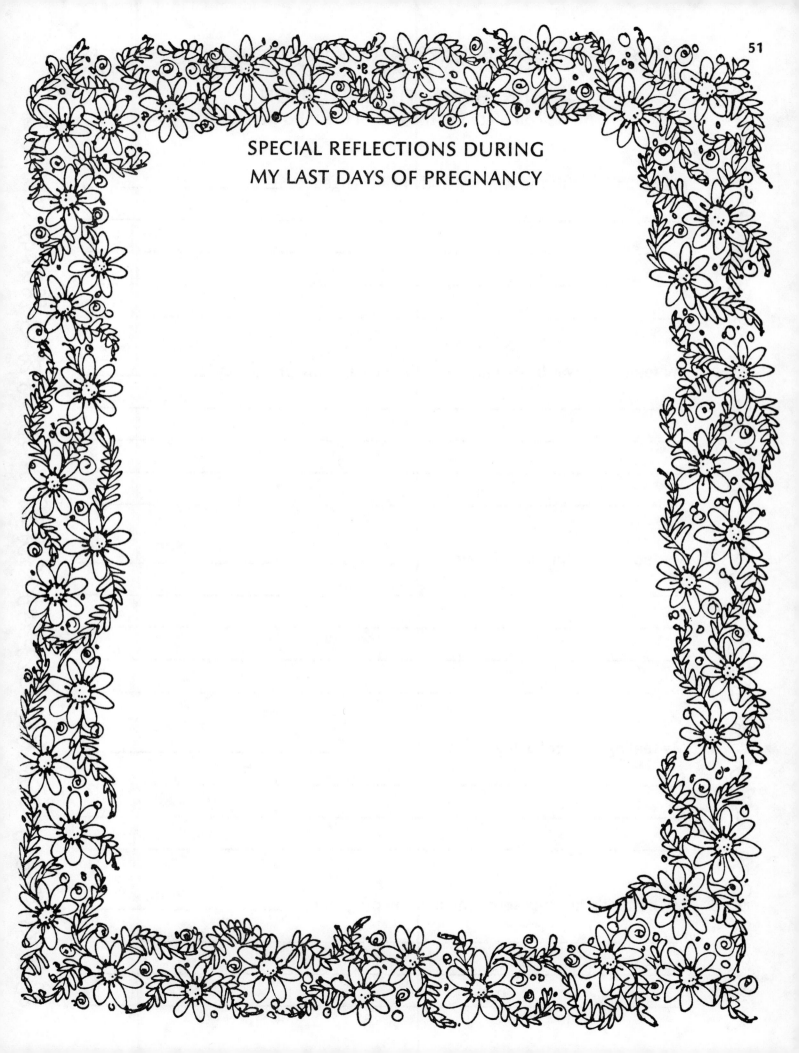

NINTH MONTH EVALUATION
(to be completed at the end of the third trimester)

1. My feelings about the way my body has changed: _____

    _____

    _____

    _____

    _____

2. My feelings towards my partner at this stage of my pregnancy: _____

    _____

    _____

    _____

    _____

3. My feelings about making love: _____

    _____

    _____

    _____

    _____

4. My feelings about having this baby: _____

    _____

    _____

    _____

5. My partner's feelings about me and my pregnancy: _____

    _____

    _____

    _____

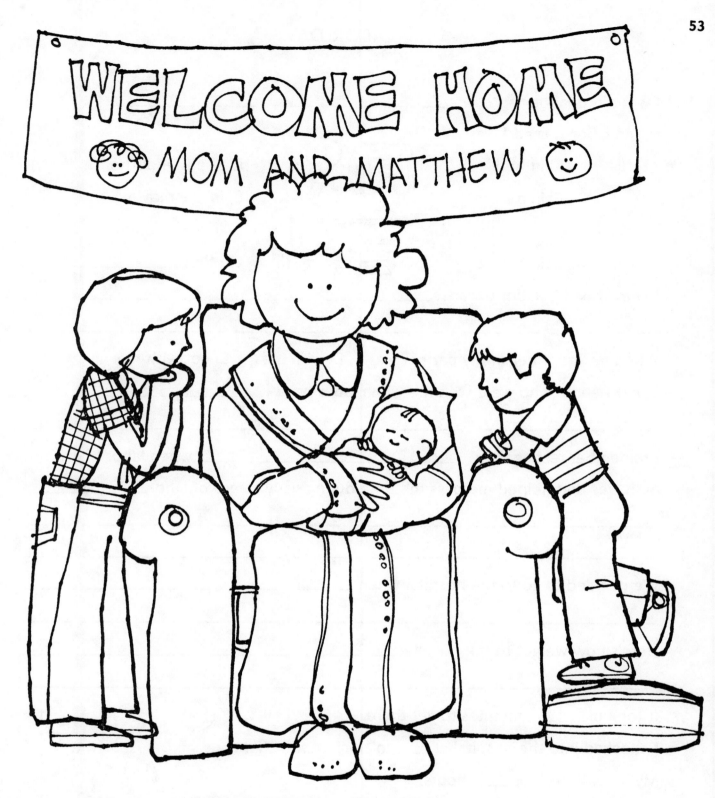

A TIME FOR CHANGE....

LABOR DAY

I went into labor on _____ _____ _____

When labor started I was

- ☐ in bed
- ☐ in a store
- ☐ in the bathtub
- ☐ in the car

- ☐ at a friend's house
- ☐ in the movies
- ☐ in a restaurant
- ☐ other _____

I knew I was in labor because_____

_____

When my labor began my partner was   ☐ with me   ☐ not with me.

Other people who were with me when labor began _____

_____

I remember feeling very _____when labor began.

Activities that helped me pass the time during early stages of labor_____

_____

_____

We decided to go to the hospital when _____

_____

Here's how we got to the hospital_____

_____

It took us_____minutes to get there.

I checked into the hospital at_____o'clock A.M.   P.M.

My labor lasted for_____hours.

My overall impressions of the hospital and staff during labor _____

_____

_____

_____

A BLOW BY BLOW DESCRIPTION OF BIRTH

My early contractions came every____minutes and lasted for_____. When I entered the hospital, I was already dilated to_____cm.

Some of the things that helped me during the first stage of labor up to the pushing stage _____

_____

_____

Some of the things that hindered me _____

_____

_____

I recognized I was in transition because _____

_____

_____

In the harder or more active stage of my labor, my contractions came every_____ minutes and lasted for _____.

I pushed for _____.

My baby was born at _____O'clock A.M. P.M.

I had the following: ☐I.V.   ☐Glucose   ☐Episiotomy   ☐Fetal Monitor

☐Pitocin   ☐Ultrasound   ☐Amniocentisis   ☐X-rays

I had the following medications: _____

My overall experience of birth compared to my expectations_____

_____

_____

The one thing I'd like to be different next time _____

_____

_____

FOR CAESAREAN MOTHERS

I had a C-birth because _____

_____

_____

I ____ did ____ did not know I was having a C-birth in advance.

My reactions and feelings about having a C-birth _____

_____

_____

I learned about C-births through:

_____classes   _____friends

_____films   _____my doctor

_____books   _____other

The person who was most supportive during the operation was_____

_____

My partner ____ was ____ was not with me during the birth.

Type of anesthesia used: _____

MY FEELINGS

I was surprised that _____

_____

The best part_____

_____

The worst part _____

_____

I was relieved that _____

_____

I first saw my baby _____

I first held my baby _____

FIRST IMPRESSIONS

My first thoughts and feelings after seeing my baby:

My thoughts and feelings about the delivery:

I first held my baby when_____

My feelings about holding my baby for the first time:

I first heard my baby cry when: _____

My feelings about hearing my baby cry for the first time:

I first nursed or fed my baby when _____

My thoughts and feelings about feeding my baby for the first time:

My feelings about being a mother:

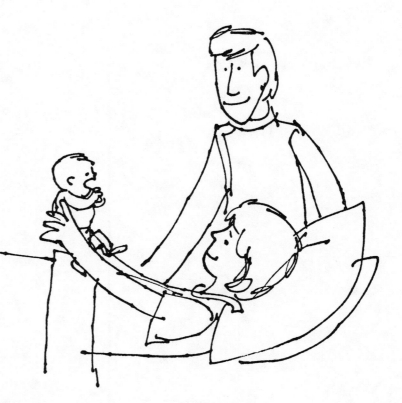

FATHER'S VIEW

Here is my partner's account of the birth of our child.

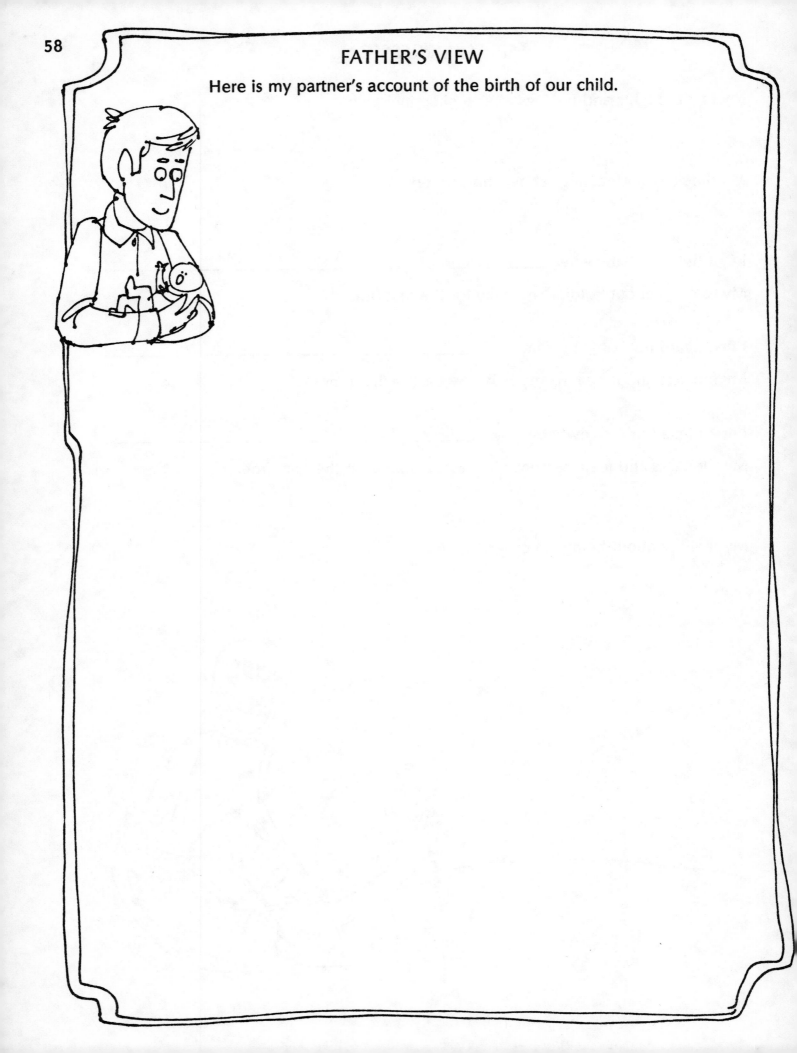

The first people I called after the delivery _____

_____

_____

Here's what happened right after the delivery:

I ____ did ____ did not have rooming-in.

My feelings about the hospital arrangements for my baby and myself:

Special calls and visitors:

Comments on my hospital stay:

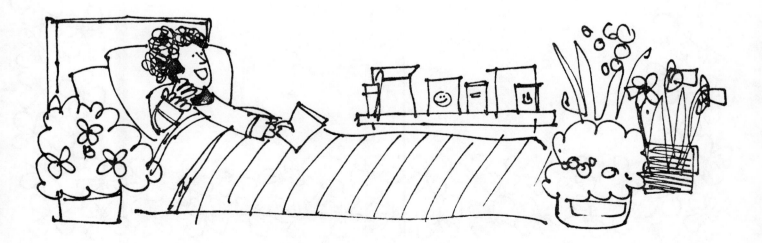

MY OWN EXPERIENCE

Thoughts and reflections on my child's birth.

MY OWN EXPERIENCE, continued

HOMECOMING DAY

I left the hospital on _____ at _____ o'clock after a _____ day stay.

Here is what I wore _____

Here is what my baby wore_____

_____

Here's how we got home _____

_____ was waiting to greet us at home.

The best part about being home is _____

_____

_____

The worst part about being home is_____

_____

_____

_____ is planning to help me at home with the baby.

Some special things I want to remember about the day we brought our baby home _____

_____

_____

_____

_____

_____

FATHER'S REFLECTIONS

I celebrated fatherhood by _____

_____

When I first held my baby I_____

_____

My greatest surprise was _____

_____

I think the best part about being a father will be_____

_____

I think the most difficult part of fatherhood for me will be _____

_____

Plans I have for myself as a father: _____

_____

_____

_____

_____

PORTRAITS OF BABY

Comments! Drawings! Opinions! Impressions! Reactions
by family and friends who came to visit.

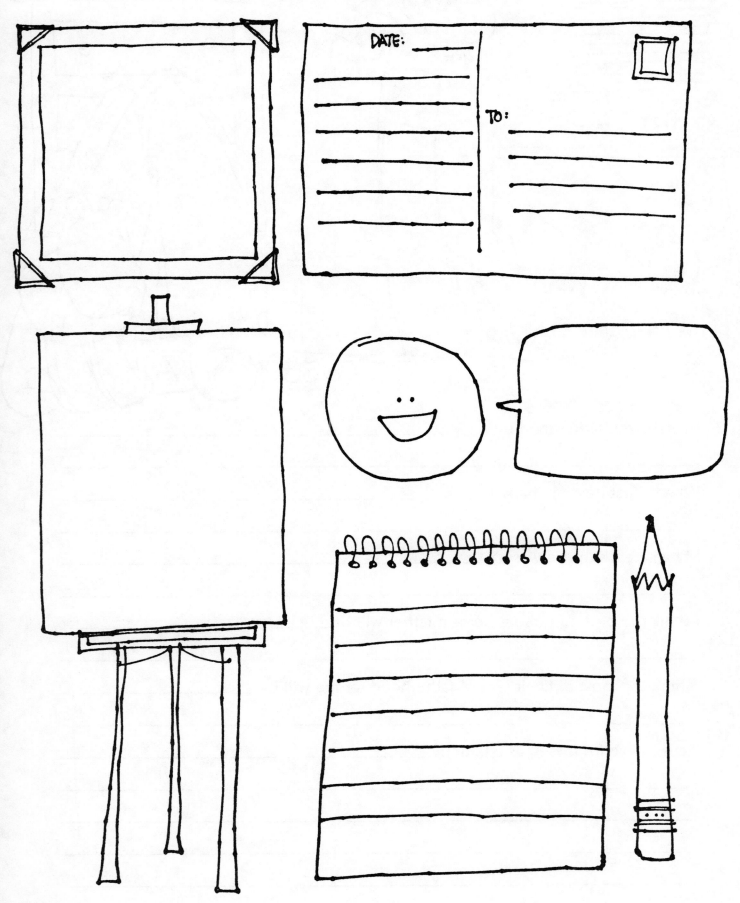

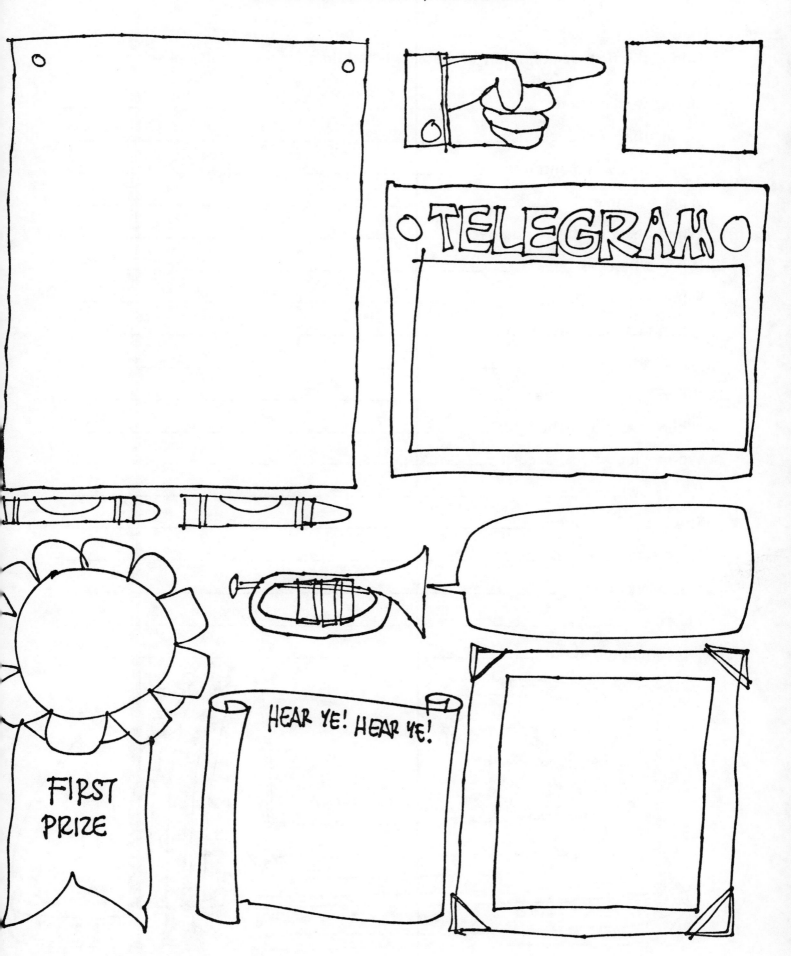

TELEGRAM

FIRST PRIZE

HEAR YE! HEAR YE!

GETTING ACQUAINTED

During the first week home with baby I've had time for these quick observations:

During feeding time: _____

During diaper changes: _____

When uncovered and free: _____

What s/he likes: _____

When being washed or bathed _____

When s/he cries: _____

When s/he sleeps: _____

When hearing a new noise: _____

When riding in the car: _____

When I talk to him/her: _____

When seeing a bright light: _____

When a loud noise occurs: _____

It took awhile: _____

The baby discovered: _____

I'm greatly relieved: _____

I'm surprised that: _____

I like: _____

I'm concerned about: _____

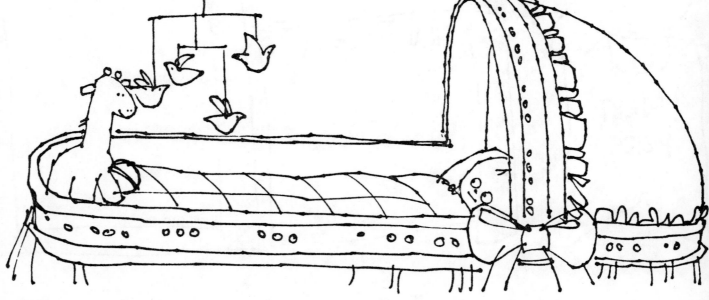

A PERSONALITY OF HIS/HER OWN

During the first few weeks of living with and observing_____, I have found

that he/she has her own unique style. Circle one from each.

More like a tennis racket or a tennis ball?

More like a clock or a sundial?

More like a locked cabinet or a barn door?

More like the river or the dam?

More like a rock band or a string quartet?

More like tickling or back scratching?

More like half-full or half-empty?

More like here or there?

More like a tortoise or a hare?

More like a novel or a comic strip?

More like the sun or the moon?

HERE

THERE

THE GREAT AMERICAN BABY

THE CHARTREUSE CACAPHONY

REFLECTIONS

NOW THAT MY PREGNANCY IS OVER, HERE ARE SOME PERSONAL THOUGHTS AND FEELINGS ABOUT MY EXPERIENCE.

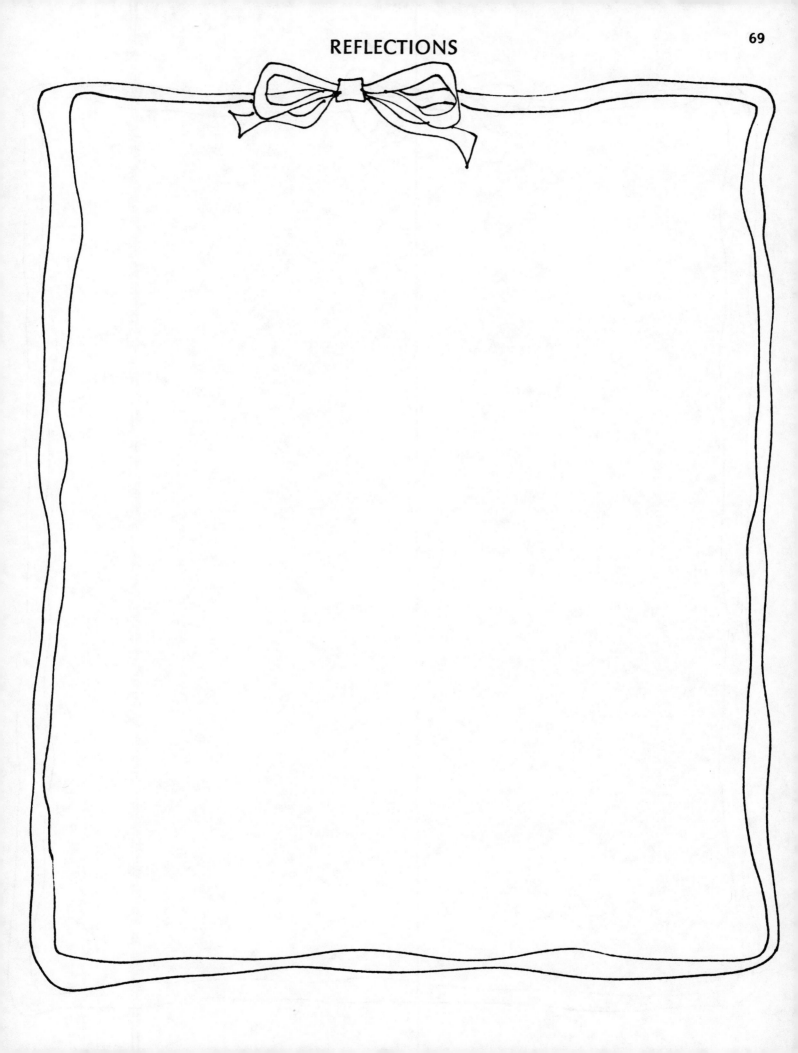

REFLECTIONS

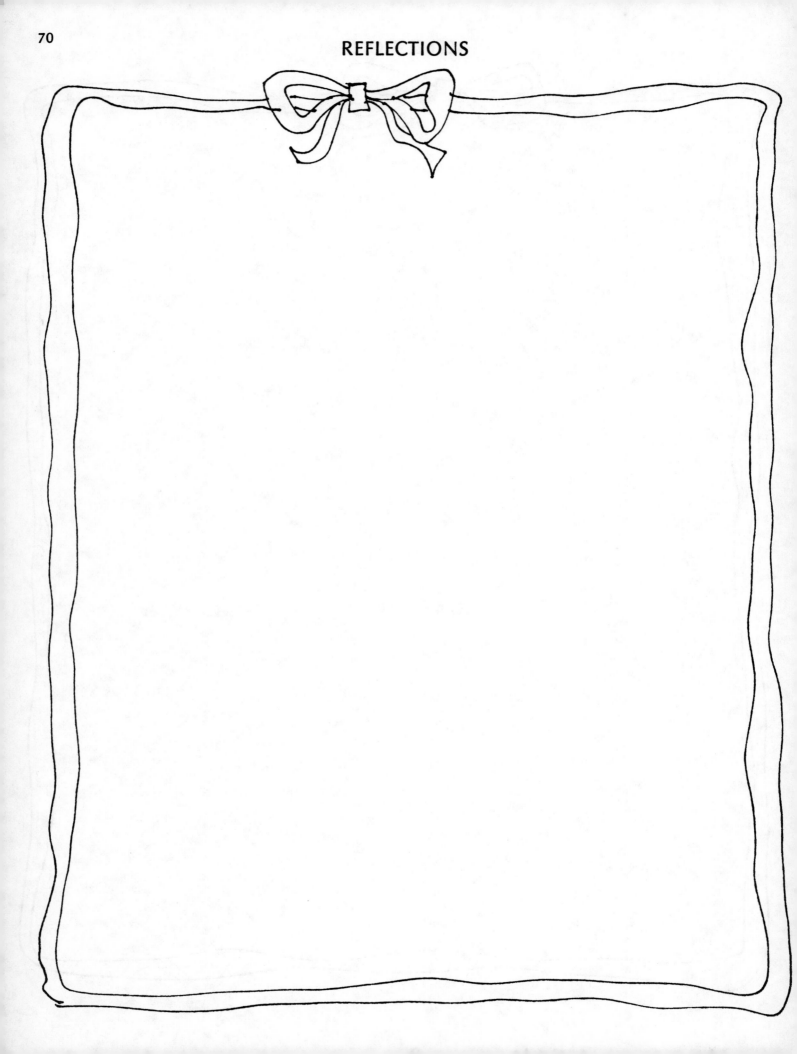

REFLECTIONS

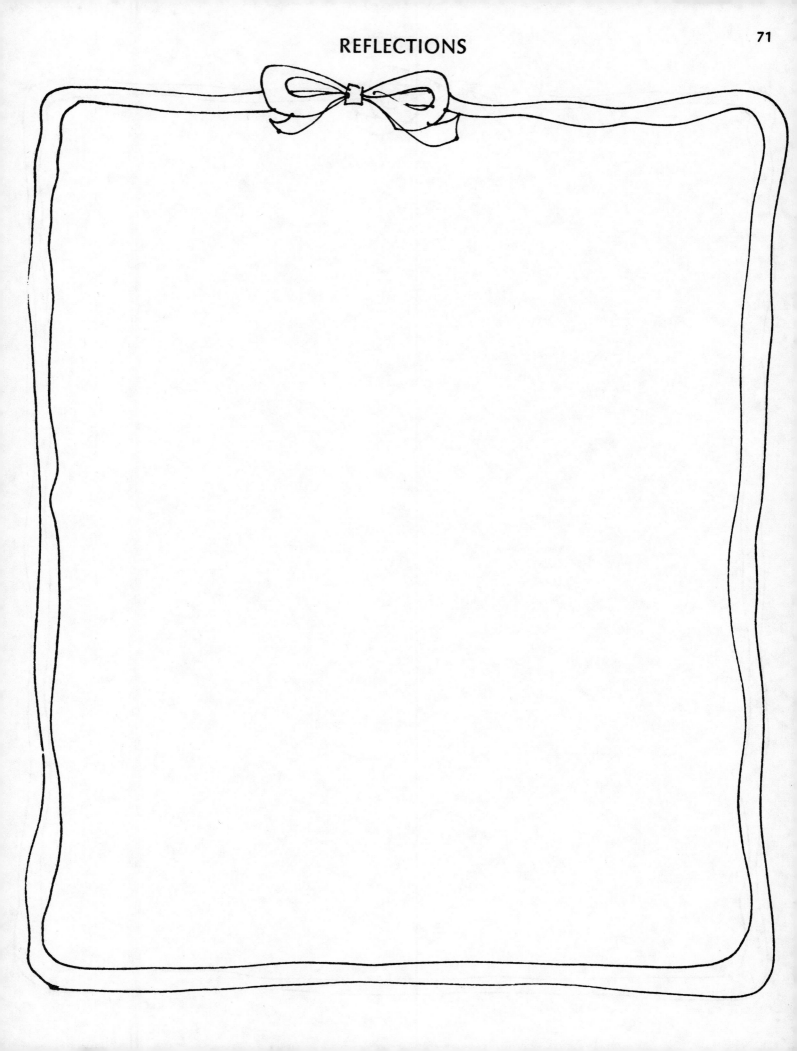

REFLECTIONS

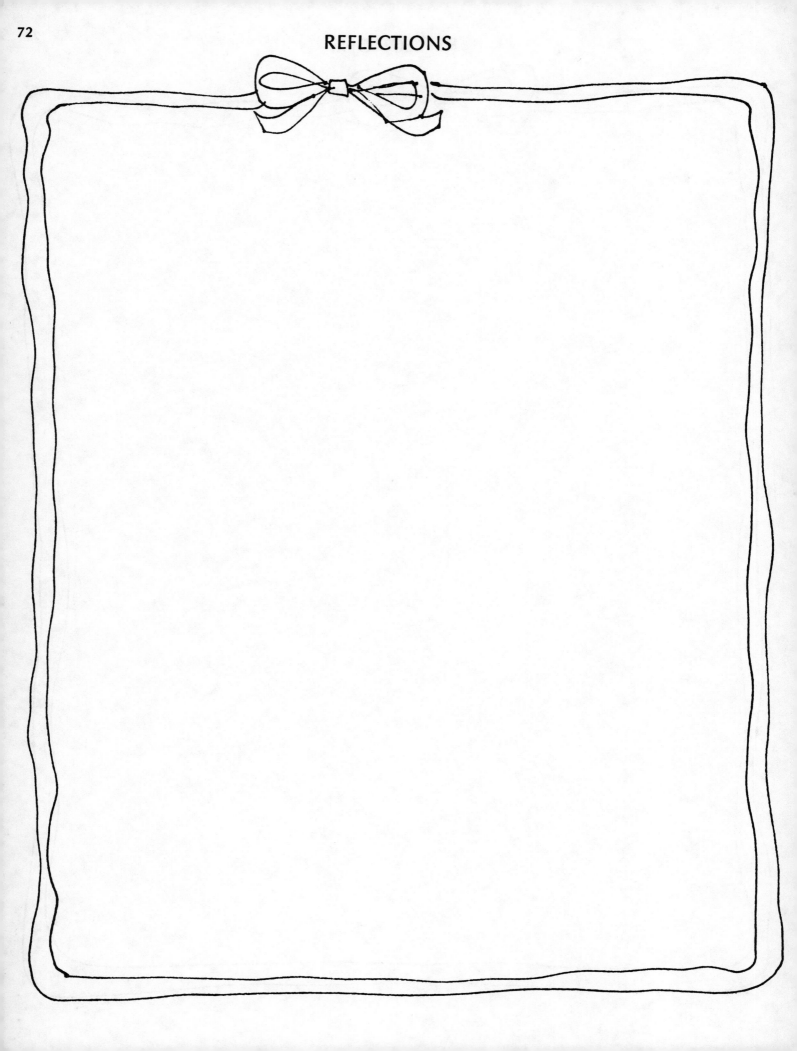

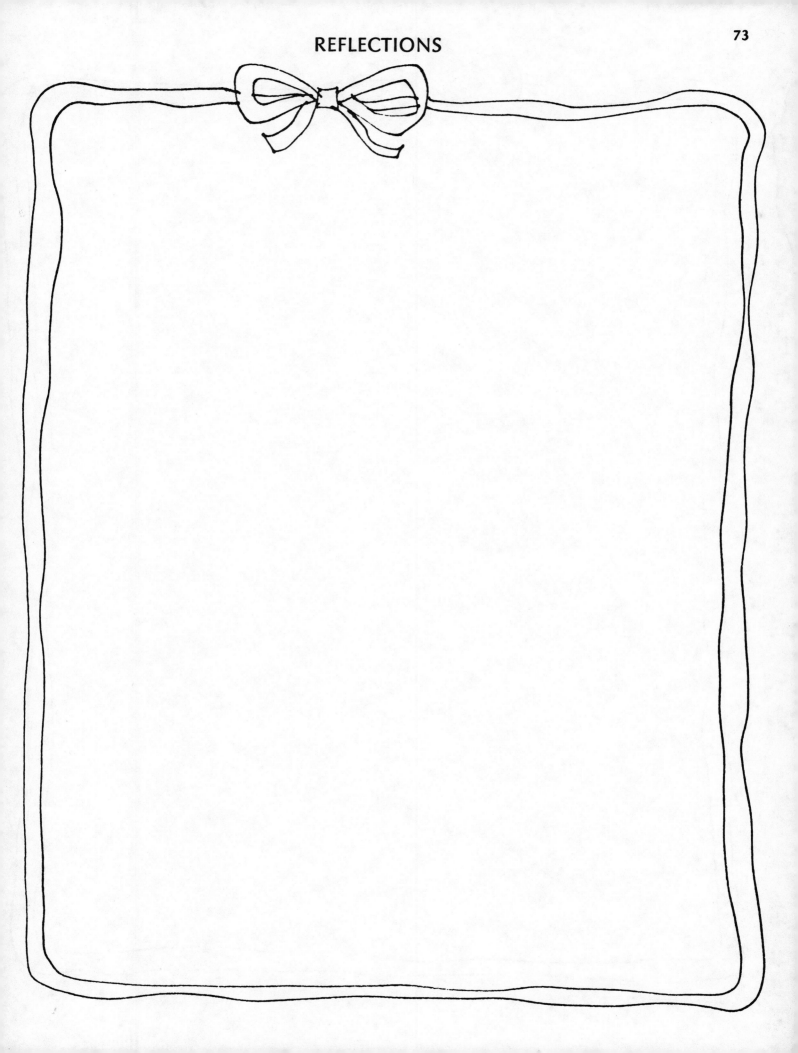

REFLECTIONS

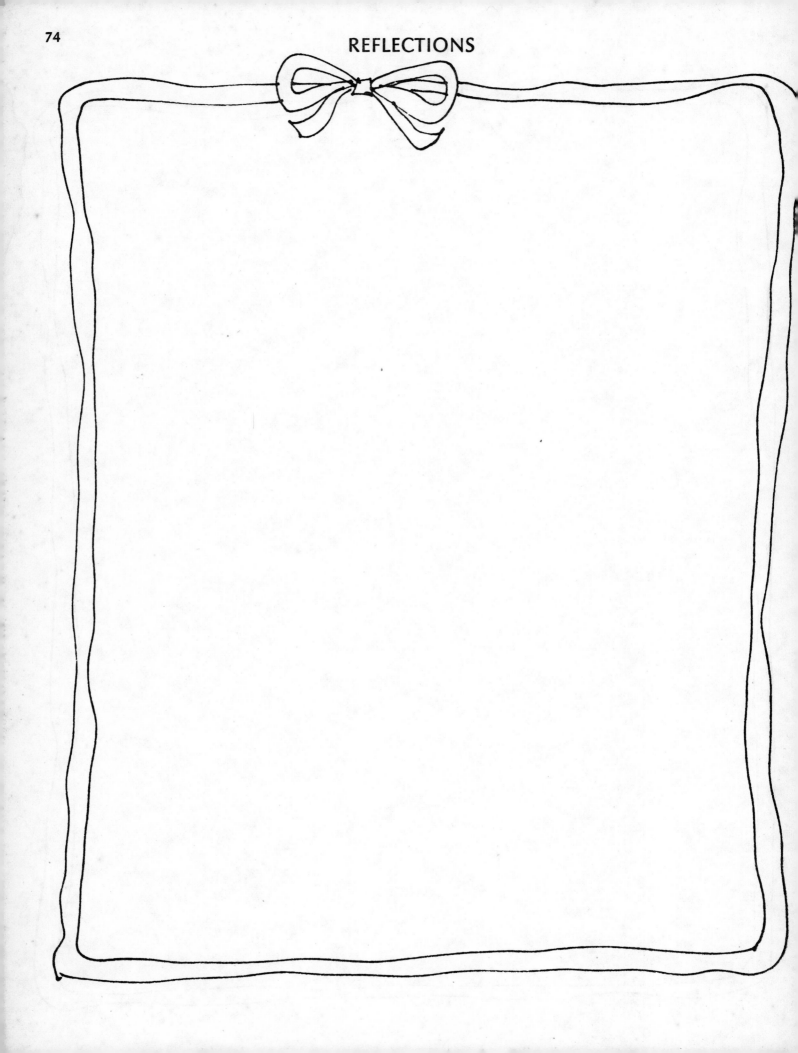